Hot & Cold Stone Massage Therapy:

A Guide to the Total Mind-Body Experience

Ernesto Ortiz LMT, CST

Mud Puddle inc.
NEW YORK

Hot & Cold Stone Massage Therapy:
A Guide to the Total Mind-Body Experience
by Ernesto Ortiz LMT, CST

Copyright ©2009 by Mud Puddle Books, Inc.

Published by
Mud Puddle, Inc.
36 W. 25th Street
5th Floor
New York, NY 10010
info@mudpuddleinc.com

ISBN: 978-1-60311-198-0

Photographic credits: Ernesto Ortiz

Design by Amy Trombat

Printed in China

....

Please note:
Not all massage techniques are appropriate for everyone, especially
those with back problems or other physical disorders. To reduce the
risk of potential injury, be sure to consult with your doctor before
beginning this or any other massage program.

The creators, producers, participants and distributors of this program
disclaim any liability or loss in connection with the Hot Stone
Massage and general massage techniques contained in this program.

This program is for private non-professional use only.

Contents

Introduction *5*

1 The Ancient Use of Stones *8*

2 The Stones We Use *10*

3 The Unseen World of Stones *12*

4 Chakras *14*

5 Supplies *19*

6 Stone Placement in Roaster *23*

7 Cold Stone Storage *25*

8 Temperature Settings *26*

Preparing Hot Stones

Preparing Cold Stones

9 Trouble Shooting Tips *28*

If the stones are too hot…

If the stones are not hot enough…

If your partner says that the applied stones are too hot…

If your partner says that the stones in your hand are too hot…

10 Thermotherapy *31*

Reflex Effects of Prolonged Cold

Reflex Effects Produced by Alternating Hot & Cold

Reflex Effects of Prolonged Heat

Hydrostatic Effect

Active Hyperemia

Indications for Cold

Indications for Heat

11   Benefits of the Application of Stones Over… *37*

      Hands

      Feet

      Heart area

      Lungs

      Stomach

      Kidneys

      Muscles

      Nervous System

12   Contrast Local Applications *39*

13   Using Hot & Cold Stones *41*

14   Terminology *42*

15   Stone Layouts *44*

16   Basic Hot Stone Treatment *46*

17   Additional Stone Layouts *60*

18   House Calls *63*

     About the Author *64*

Introduction

I WOULD LIKE TO WELCOME YOU TO A WONDERFUL adventure of self-exploration and intimacy, an adventure that can be shared with a loved one, partner or a friend.

What I am going to share with you will open you and your partner to a new type of sensory adventure.

I recommend that before you enter into massage practice you read this book from cover to cover so you have the basic understanding of the techniques employed. It wouldn't hurt to read this book more than once so you can have greater knowledge of the principles contained.

A hot stone massage session has been described in many ways: delicious, decadent, sensual, totally relaxing, and deeply therapeutic; a moving experience, comforting, and, above all, healing.

This experience has the ability to positively affect your four lower bodies. The four lower bodies are the mental, emotional, physical and spiritual. These provide the way we express and relate to the world. We utilize one or two more than the others but it is inevitable that we utilize all of them to experience life. Each body functions separately but at the same time they unite to give life expression.

As you learn to prepare the stones you will see how we use the basic elements of life, fire, water, air and earth to create our session. When we overlap the four lower bodies (mental, emotional, physical and spiritual) with the basic elements that create life (fire, water, air and earth) we end up with a powerful combination that has all of the ingredients to promote change.

The way these elements relate to each other is:

Fire is in direct relation to the spiritual body.
Water is in direct relation to the emotional body.
Air is in direct relation to the mental body.
Earth is in direct relation to the physical body.

This combination makes hot stone massage a total healing experience that you can share with your friends and loved ones.

This book is the result of over 12 years of teaching thousands of Licensed Massage Therapists and having a private practice utilizing hot and cold stones as tools for change and transformation. It is my desire to share this with you so you have the same opportunity to make a positive impact not only on your life but the life of the one you share the technique with.

I have heard the effect of hot stone massage described in many ways: extremely balancing, delicious, like going back to the womb, deeply connecting, freed me from my muscular restrictions, I felt like melted chocolate. In other words, once you become accomplished at it, you will provide an experience like no other.

Be open to explore, be open to experience and to feel new sensations, and allow the stones to bring a new kinds of pleasures and sensations into your life.

Let the adventure begin!
Ernesto

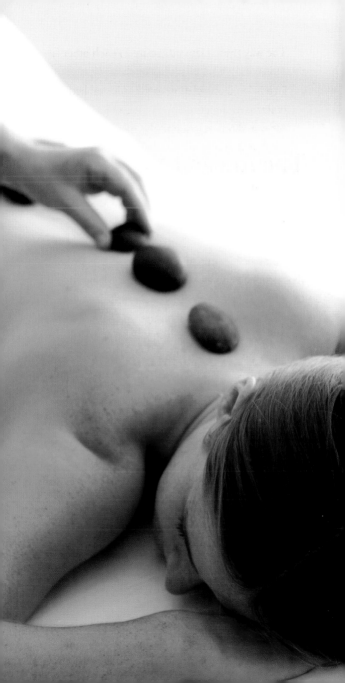

1

The Ancient Use of Stones

MAN'S USE OF STONES GOES BACK LONG BEFORE recorded history. Even a cursory look at ancient cultures and civilizations reveals the importance of stones. At a very basic level hot stones were used for heating human homes and they were an essential element in sacred rituals.

Stones were prized building material in the construction of temples and pyramids; some have stood the test of time and still amaze us today in the form of mysterious structures circling the globe from Egypt to South America, from Easter Island to the remnants of Native American cultures.

When we think of landmarks such as the pyramids or Stonehenge, we think of huge stone structures, the very construction of which seems miraculous. But smaller stones have been part of ritual and ceremony throughout history. Homes have been made of stone since before modern memory as have weapons and the tools used to sharpen them. The popularity of quartz crystals covers the entire span of human existence down to this very day, and even the non-believer or skeptic may wear a birthstone ring as a symbol of good fortune.

Native Americans have used hot stones in their sweat lodge ceremonies since ancient times. In fact, nearly twenty years ago it was this particular use that introduced me to the possibilities of using hot stones for therapy. At first I found I had a budding and growing respect for *grandfather's stones* as they are called, long before I had an understanding of the use and application of the stones to the body.

It all began with a preparation of the stones for a ritual, a preparation that incorporated all four elements— fire, water, air and earth. During this time my spiritual grandmother Barrett Eagle Bear, a Lakota medicine woman (shaman), would pass a perfectly round hot stone around the circle of participants. She would ask us to rub that stone anywhere we felt pain or discomfort on our bodies. While the stone was passed, Grandmother Barrett would tell us the story of the stone and how it got so round with the help of ants pushing and rolling it toward the river. This particular stone was given to her by her grandfather. This was my introduction to stone massage.

Today, in a world governed by ever-increasing speed and technology, we still have the opportunity to take-in and use some of the ancient rituals in modern day practice. We begin, as people have for thousands of years, with respect and reverence for the stones and to the people who have gone before us.

2

The Stones We Use

BASALT IS THE MOST COMMON VARIETY OF volcanic rock, composed almost entirely of dark, fine-grained silicate or quartz-like minerals. Because it contains different types of minerals, basalt is capable of holding heat and cold. This makes it the ideal stone for hot stone massage.

Once the stones are oiled they change in color from a dull grey to a beautiful dark color. Many times an oiled stone has shades of many other colors, an indication of the different minerals that make-up basalt. You may see steaks or lines of white which is the silica composition, or you may see deep red spots or specks which is the iron content, or green specs which is the olivine. All of these are different minerals that form basalt.

Basalt is formed by the outpouring of volcanic lava which is, as you may well know, hot and liquid- like, so hot that it cuts grooves on the earth as it follows the downhill slope of the volcano. As the hot lava flows, it picks up minerals from the earth, and as it does that, the cooling process begins. Thousands of years may pass as these basalt stones sit on river beds being washed and polished by water and friction from other stones.

Geologists measure all stones and minerals using an international measurement scale known as the Mohs scale. I am sure you have heard that a diamond is the hardest of all stones. This means that a diamond measures 10 on the Mohs scale. Basalt measures between 7.5 and 8 on the Mohs scale, making it a very hard stone. This is one of the reasons why it holds heat and cold as well as it does, and that is why it is ideal for hot stone massage.

Stone charging layout

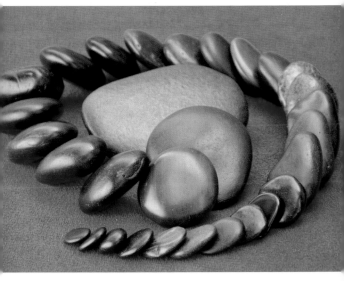

3

The Unseen World
of Stones

LEARNING EXPERIENCES ARE CLASSIFIED AS either intellectual or experiential. Intellectual experience comes from books and other written materials as well as from listening to experts. The latter may be delivered in a multitude of ways, i.e. in the form of lectures or discussions. Intellectual experience may also come from what we see, i.e. great works of art or documentaries. In short, intellectual experience depends on the dispensing of knowledge by others.

On the other hand, knowledge achieved through experiential experience is based on the examination and reflection of what one has done by one's own self. In other words, experiential experience is the primary learning process for any individual. If, for example, we touch a hot stove, we pull back our hand and learn not to touch hot stoves. We don't have to read about this experience or listen to the experience of others; we learn by doing and then thinking about what we've done.

While it will no doubt be beneficial to read through this manual before you start working with hot and cold stones, you will find that the best way to begin is experiential. When you place stones in a roaster, you'll find that you begin to tune into their frequencies (the energy or energies emanating from the stones), first by their placement in the roaster, then by using them on yourself and by experimenting with them.

Yes, it's possible to become technically proficient in administering hot and cold massages, but this is a mechanical, passionless way of going about the work. You'll find that you achieve a greater degree of success if you tune-in to the energy of the person you're massaging. Only in this way will your partner be truly served.

We can all readily acknowledge the world of the seen. But when you're dealing with an individual's energy or, if you will, aura, you're into the world of the unseen. It takes just a little bit of creativity and imagination to picture this world populated by spirits and guides, even angels and fairies. This unseen world is certainly the abiding place of intuition, that special frequency within ourselves that allow us to hear our inner voices.

When you acknowledge the energy of the stones and truly imagine the elements that go into their preparation, you will find it easy to look on their effects as a ritual of nature, fire, air and earth. By using your intuition, you'll find it possible to connect these elements to the stones, and always remember to allow your intuition to play an important role in hot and cold stone massage. The more you use your intuition and the more you know the stones, the deeper you can get into your work.

4

Chakras

WITHIN THE SPIRITUAL REALM OF EVERY
living body, there are a series of energy fields very
much like generators. These fields are called chakras.
These energy centers have been known to Asian cultures
for more than 2,000 years, but it's only in the last few
decades that this information has been widely circulated
in the west.

The word Chakra is Sanskrit for "wheel." Chakras
are conceptualized as spinning wheels, as you can see in
the illustration (p. 17) showing the energy centers located
within the body, in front and back of the spinal column.

Each chakra has a color and vibrates to a specific
frequency. By using stones in the front and back of the
body, we address these centers of energy. We can both
directly and indirectly energize and balance the chakras
with the assistance of the stones.

The major Chakra centers are:

The numbers correspond to the numbers on the diagram on page 17

1

Base, or Root Chakra

Location: Base of the spine

Color: Red

This is the chakra closest to the earth. It represents our grounding to the earth and to the physical plane.

2

Sacral, or Naval Chakra

Location: Between the base of the spine and the navel

Color: Orange

This chakra represents our sexuality, including our sexual impulses, and our creativity.

3

Solar Plexus

Location: The solar plexus area about 2" (5cm) below the navel

Color: Yellow

The solar plexus is the seat of personal emotions, which include feelings of personal power, anger and hostility. Our intuition is stored here, and it can be said that the solar plexus is the center of psychic (etheric) intuition. This is the seat of our emotional life, hence the age-old reference to "gut feeling."

4

Heart

Location: Center of chest

Color: Green

The heart is the center of love, harmony and peace. It is the place of union between the upper and lower chakras. It is through the heart that we find love, which then travels to the emotional center (the Solar Plexus), then to the Sacral Chakra which adds strong feelings of attraction and passion, and then to the Root Chakra which promotes the feelings of wanting to settle down. The love energies that have traveled down to the Base (root) move up again to the Heart and to the Crown for complete union.

5

Throat

Location: Within the throat

Color: Blue

This is the center of communication, self-expression and judgment. Should you experience any problems with communication, you can draw the color blue to this area, and it will help you say what needs to be said.

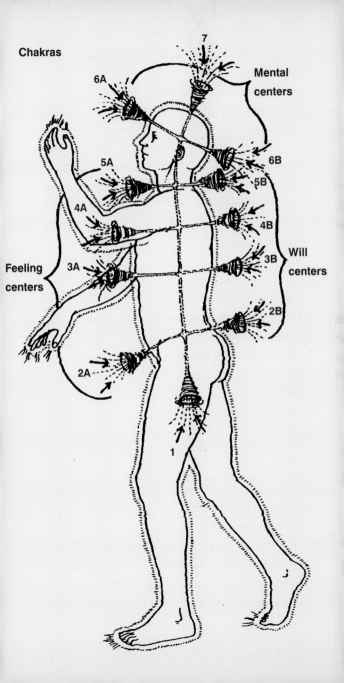

Third Eye, or Brow Chakra
Location: Center of the forehead
Color: Indigo

This chakra is used to question the spiritual nature of our lives. Our inner vision is contained here as well as inner gifts of clairvoyance, wisdom and perception. The vision and dreams of our lives are held in this chakra.

7

Crown
Location: Top of the head
Color: Violet

This is the chakra of divine purpose, the chakra of destiny. It is the doorway to the divine and the transpersonal (the areas of consciousness beyond personal identity) chakras. It balances our interior with our exterior and brings them into a harmonious voice.

8, 9, 10 etc.

Transpersonal Chakras

These are our true connections with the divine as well as the connections between masters and teachers. We experience grace, ecstasy and spiritual union with God from these chakras.

5

Supplies

Here is a list of supplies that you will need to perform hot and cold stone massage.

Basalt Stones

As you choose your stones for massage, you need to look for stones that fit your hands comfortably while also considering the application of that stone. The edges must be smooth and round and the size will vary according to the use from small quarter-size stones for the toes to large effleurage stones. Medium effleurage stones can also be used cold.

Roasters

The roaster is the most essential tool other than the stones. Roasters are the best way to heat up the stones. An 8-quart

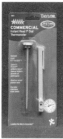

(7.5L) roaster is ideal for our work.

Thermometer

An essential tool! The water in the roaster is heated to 135°F to 138°F (57°C to 59°C). To monitor the water temperature for an hour or longer you will need an accurate thermometer. Look in hardware stores for the best kind. Meat thermometers work well. Candy thermometers are not as accurate. Thermometers should range from 0°F to 160°F (-18°C to 71°C).

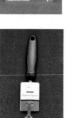

Spoon

You will need a wooden spoon to remove the stones from the roaster. I use a large slotted wood spoon so the water can drain.

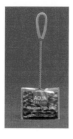

Bag and Net

You are going to need one 4" (10cm) aquarium fish net with a long handle to hold the toe stones. You'll also need one small laundry bag (the type used for hosiery and delicates). This bag is for the spinal layout stones.

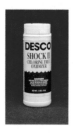

Spa Oxidizer

This is going to help keep the water sanitized and the roaster clean throughout the day. At the end of the day you will need to wash your stones and roaster with warm

Spinal layout

6

Stone Placement in Roaster

WHEN PLACING STONES IN THE ROASTER, YOU'LL find it best to develop a system of placement. This will help avoid confusion and wasted time. In an accompanying drawing, you'll find an easy-to-use, easy-to-remember suggestion for the placing of the stones.

Stand facing the front of the roaster. Imagine the roaster as a clock, its center being where the hands of the clock meet. In the center stack the Sacral and Belly Stones. Directly above at 12 o'clock, place four large effleurage stones.

At one o'clock, stack six neck stones.

Below that, at four or five o'clock, stack two hand stones.

At six o'clock, stack four large effleurage stones.

In massage therapy effleurage is a term indicating long, gliding strokes, and effleurage stones are the stones used for this. These strokes may be used to connect one body part with another, i.e., the transition from the legs to the back is done by gliding with a long effleurage stroke.

At eight, nine and ten o'clock, stack the medium effleurage stones.

The spinal layout stones, which are in a net bag, should be placed on top of the medium effleurage stones on the left hand side of the roaster.

Finally, the toe, eye and throat chakra stones should be placed in a net on top of the neck stones on the right hand side of the roaster.

If this set-up doesn't work for you, develop a system for yourself that is both comfortable and practical. Whatever works for you is the correct way to go.

Stone Placement in Roaster

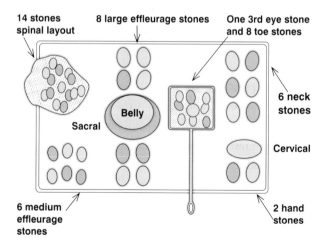

Front of Roaster

7

Cold Stone Storage

I SUGGEST KEEPING COLD STONES IN A FREEZER at all times so that they are always ready when needed.

When you move the stones from the freezer to the massage room, transport them in an ice chest containing several frozen ice packs to keep the stones cold.

If a freezer isn't handy, use a small ice chest filled halfway with ice. The stones should be placed on top of the ice until cold. Usually it takes about an hour for the stones to be ready.

The proper way to transport the stones from the ice chest to the massage site is to place the stones on a towel. This will prevent the stones from dripping when applied to your partner.

8

Temperature Settings

Preparing Hot Stones

Place a hand towel at the bottom of the roaster to cushion the stones. Then place the stones in the roaster with just enough hot water to cover them. Hot water from the faucet is usually delivered between 115°F to 120°F (46°C to 49°C). By using the roaster, you're able to adjust the temperature of the water as needed.

Raise the temperature of the water to about 135°F to 140°F (57°C to 60°C). At this temperature the stones will sit comfortably in your hands and will be in the range that most partners tolerate very well (this range is generally between 135°F to 138°F [57°C to 59°C]; ideally, 135°F [57°C]).

Constantly check your thermometer and adjust the temperature according to your needs. For example, you will most likely have to raise the temperature after you finish the front of the body to get the stones hot again before beginning to work on the back.

Tip: add a few drops of essential oil to the water before the treatment. Your partner will be greeted by a pleasingly fragrant room.

Preparing Cold Stones

Preparation is particularly simple: place the cold stones in a small ice chest which is half-filled with ice and you're ready to go.

Cold stones work very well on areas of recent injuries, burns and inflammation. In addition, I have found that the use of cold stones after the use of hot stones is particularly effective in the shoulder and neck areas. Partners love the contrast.

Remember that iced stones penetrate far deeper than hot stones, so it's important not to keep the cold stones in one area too long. It's possible to burn your partner with cold as well as hot stones.

Back chakra layout

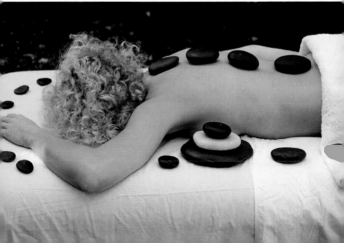

9

Trouble Shooting Tip

If the stones are too hot:

1. Check the temperature of the roaster. If the temperature is too high, replace some of the hot water with cold.
2. You can cool the stones with alcohol or dunk them in a small bucket of cold water for approximately five seconds.
3. Set the stones out on a towel until they cool to the desired temperature.

If the stones are not hot enough:

1. Check the temperature of the roaster and increase the temperature as needed.
2. Continue to massage your partner while waiting for the water to heat up.
3. To speed the heating process, cover the roaster.

If your partner says that the applied stones are too hot:

1. If all the stones are too hot, use an additional pillow-case.

   You'll need three pillowcases: one is placed directly on top of the massage table to prevent the vinyl from damage from the repetitive use of hot stones on the sheet covering the massage table; the second pillowcase and the third, if necessary, cover the stones to prevent the hot stones from burning your partner.

2. If one or two stones are reported to be too hot, add another layer to these stones. *Tip:* children's socks usually work well for wrapping individual stones. In any case, it's always best to have additional fabric on hand in case your partner is too sensitive to the heat.

If your partner says that the stones in your hands are too hot:

1. Be aware of each individual's sensitivity to heat. If your partner says the stones in your hand are too hot and the water in the roaster is at the right temperature, lower the temperature to 125°F to 130°F (52°C to 54°C).
2. Leave the stones out of the roaster to cool for a few minutes while you continue to massage. Then reapply the stones.
3. Make certain that you are applying the right amount of pressure to your partner's body.

❖ Firm pressure that goes below the skin is the best pressure to use.

❖ Be careful: a light massage with a hot stone will burn your partner.

❖ Keep the stones moving. Do not hold a stationary hot stone on a body part; this will burn your partner, especially if the stones are fresh out of hot water.

Gliding stroke or Effleurage stroke

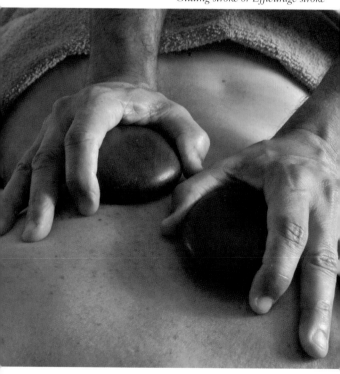

10

Thermotherapy

STONE MASSAGE IS BASED ON THE PRINCIPLE OF thermotherapy. Scientifically, the definition of thermotherapy is: the application of either hot or cold to the body for the purpose of changing the physiological responses that are going on in the body. In other words, we use hot and cold massage to promote healing, balance and well-being.

While there are many styles of massage available today, no massage has proven to be more effective than hot and cold massage in promoting a state of "homeostasis," which is a state of perfect equilibrium within the body. When the body has reached a desired state of stability, psychological tension is reduced and often eliminated.

Further, with the use of hot and cold stones, circulation is rapidly altered. When circulation increases, so does the delivery of nutrition to every cell in the body. Increased blood flow also motivates the body to detoxify, therefore promoting healing.

The application of either hot or cold stones produces a series of internal responses:

1. Depletion: This is the withdrawal of blood and lymph from one area to another caused by the simultaneous application of stones to different body areas.

2. Prolonged application of hot stones to an area acts as a derivative. This is the decreasing of blood and lymph from one area by increasing blood and lymph in another resulting in a greater amount of circulation and detoxification at the same time. The opposite effect occurs with a short application of cold stones (this is called retrostasis, the pushing of lymph and blood).

By understanding these responses, you will be able to best determine the course of treatment to your partner.

Reflex Effects of Prolonged Cold

1. Prolonged cold over an artery produces a contraction of the artery and its surrounding area.
2. Prolonged cold over the nose and the back of the neck causes the contraction of the blood vessels of the nose.
3. Prolonged cold over the abdomen causes an increase

of blood flow to promote digestive activity.

4. Prolonged cold over acute inflamed joints or bursae (the fluid sacs which prevent friction at joints, tendons, ligaments and bones) causes constriction of the blood vessels and relief of pain.

5. Prolonged cold over areas of acute trauma such as contusions and sprains will reduce pain and swelling.

6. The overall application of cold stones removes waste products from the body and increases the metabolic rate (the amount of energy spent while resting in a naturally temperate environment).

Reflex Effects Produced by Alternating Hot & Cold

Hyperemia is a desired state that results from the application of hot and cold together. Specifically, hyperemia is the increase of blood flow to the muscles and tissues. It is outwardly characterized by a superficial redness on the skin which is an indication that oxygen is being promoted to the muscles and tissues which, in turn, promotes healing.

Partners who suffer from chronic pain will feel tremendous relief with the application of hot and cold. Congestion and trigger points will be erased from the body.

Trigger points are areas of tenderness in a muscle, an indication of a high accumulation of toxins. There are two types of trigger points: active and latent.

Active trigger points cause muscular pain and will

send or direct (refer) pain and tenderness to another area of the body when pressure is applied.

Tenderness is apt to disappear in as few as one or two passes over a trigger point with a hot stone.

Latent trigger points only exhibit pain when compressed and do not refer pain to other areas of the body. Latent trigger points are believed to be one of the causes of stiff joints and the restriction of motion in older individuals.

Hot stone massage addresses latent trigger points and helps increase mobility in most individuals.

Reflex Effects of Long-Term Heat

1. Long-term heat to one extremity causes the dilation of blood vessels in the opposite extremity (i.e., the application of hot stones to the right leg will produce the desired effect in the left leg). This helps create a greater amount of circulation and detoxification.
2. Long-term heat to the abdomen will cause decreased internal blood flow and less acidity in the stomach.
3. Long-term heat to the chest promotes the ease of respiration and expectoration. Expectoration is the act of coughing and clearing the chest of mucus (phlegm).
4. Long-term heat promotes an increase of an individual's metabolic rate which, in turn, brings an increase of nutrition to the cells.
5. Long-term heat nurtures a greater feeling of comfort and relaxation.

Hydrostatic Effect

When a large area of the body's surface is exposed to heat, a general dilation of the blood vessels of the skin takes place. This is the body's method of eliminating heat. The shifting of fluid from one part of the body to another is often referred to as the hydrostatic effect.

Active Hyperemia

Hyperemia: An unusual amount of blood in a part. An increase in the quality of blood flowing through any part of the body, shown by the redness of the skin (definition from Taber's Medical Dictionary).

The short- and long-term application of cold therapy is called active hyperemia. The superficial constriction of the skin (short-term) and the dilation of the blood vessels of the skin (long-term) relieves congestion and blockages in both the internal organs and the muscle fibers.

Indications for Cold

- ✤ Relief of pain.
- ✤ Prevention and reduction of swelling.
- ✤ Early treatments of sprain, contusions and any type of muscle injury.

❖ Acute joint inflammation and arthritis.

Indications for Heat

❖ For the relief of localized pain.

❖ Derivation (the action of receiving) to increase blood flow in order to relieve congestion internally.

❖ To promote skin and tissue warming to produce relaxation.

❖ Sedative; in this case, the promotion of a natural calmness by using mild heat to relieve insomnia, stress and tension.

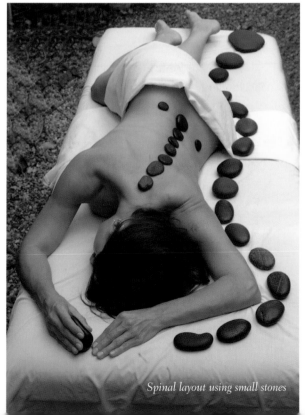

Spinal layout using small stones

11

Benefits of the Application of Stones Over...

Hands:

- ❖ Relieves arthritic and stiff joints.
- ❖ Produces general body warming.

Feet:

- ❖ Increases the blood flow through the feet and the entire skin surface.
- ❖ Helps to relieve headache pain.
- ❖ Helps to lessen chest congestion.
- ❖ Promotes a general body warming.

Heart area:

- ❖ Helps to lower blood pressure.

Lungs:

❖ Increases respiration and expectoration.

Stomach:

❖ Slows digestion and decreases gastric acidity.

Kidneys (lower back):

❖ Relieves pain due to muscle spasms.

Muscles:

❖ Softens and relaxes the muscles, increases blood flow which brings oxygen to the muscles.

Nervous System:

❖ Sedative and relaxing.

12

Contrast Local Applications

THIS IS THE ALTERNATE APPLICATION OF HOT and cold stones, usually two to three applications of hot stones to one application of cold stones.

The benefits of this are:

1. Reduces pain through the increased blood flow to the applied area.
2. Stimulates healing in local injuries.
3. Reduces swelling.
4. Relieves muscle stiffness and pain.

Indications

Do use hot and cold stone massage therapy for:

Acute inflammation, sprains, strains, bursitis, chronic tension, tennis elbow, headaches, bowel inflammation, constipation, atrophied muscles, menstrual cramps, and just for pleasure (because it feels soooooo good).

Contraindications

Do not use hot and cold stone massage therapy for:

Acute asthma, pregnancy (use hot or cold stones in isolated areas only), do not apply hot stones to the abdomen or legs, acute infections, acute cystitis, or on someone who dislikes or has an aversion to heat or cold.

Stone meditation

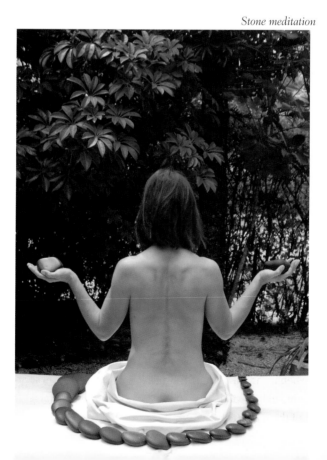

13

Using Hot & Cold Stones

THE USE OF HOT STONE IS VERY EFFECTIVE AT the beginning of a massage session, particularly if your partner suffers from chronic tension. As the session proceeds, you can add the use of cold stones as well.

If your partner is suffering from a recent sports injury, whiplash or any other type of accident, always start and finish the session by using cold stones in the particular area of the injury.

For a spinal layout, I use hot stones unless someone's back is inflamed. In that case, it's best to use cold stones over the specific area. If your partner suffers from lower back pain, you can use 4 to 6 cold stones over the lower back and hot stones for the rest of the layout.

Remember: when using cold stones, it is very important that you glide "slowly." In this way, it is much easier for your partner to tolerate the temperature of the stones. Also, when using cold stones, always tell your partner, "These are going to be cool" before applying the stones. Don't forget to tell them to breathe.

14

Terminology

A short review of the words you need to know.

Alternate: The use of hot and cold stones; a series of strokes using hot and cold stones, usually using hot stones three times more than cold stones.

Atonic: The lack of muscle tone; the lack of normal tone or strength. A reaction that shows a lessening of tone in the entire body or a specific area.

Cold stones: The use of cold stones will constrict the blood vessels while stimulating the nervous system.

Derivation: Anything derived from one part of the body to another. The drawing of blood or lymph from one part of the body using cold stones and increasing the amount of blood or lymph using hot stones in another part of the body.

Fluxion: An excessive flow or discharge from an organ of the body. An increase of blood flow resulting from the use of hot stones in an isolated area.

Hot stones: The use of hot stones will expand and dilate the blood vessels while acting as a sedative to the nervous system.

Hydrotherapy: The use of water in any of its three forms (solid, liquid or vapor) internally or externally in the treatment of disease or trauma resulting in the improvement of someone's health.

Hyperemia: An unusual amount of blood in a part of the body. An increase in the quality of blood flowing through any part of the body characterized by a redness of the skin.

Retrostasis: The pushing of blood or lymph from one area of the body to another. Use hot stones to push blood from an area where cold stones have been placed.

Tonic: An action that is invigorating and which increases strength. An action that produces a reddening of the skin (hyperemia) while increasing skin activity and respiration.

15

Stone Layouts

STONES ARE ARRANGED IN A GROUPING THAT IS in harmony with each other and not just like a pile of rocks. This harmony creates a unique energy that resonates between the stones, and this resonance keeps the electromagnetic properties of the stones charged. When the stones are in harmony this electromagnetic energy is transferred to your partner with each stroke.

Further, a stone layout is a way of keeping your stones charged and in harmony when not in use. It is a way of honoring your tools as an instrument or an extension of yourself. Creating a harmonious pattern generates a desired charge.

On page 45 you'll see some recommended stone layouts. Feel free to create your own or use the ones pictured here.

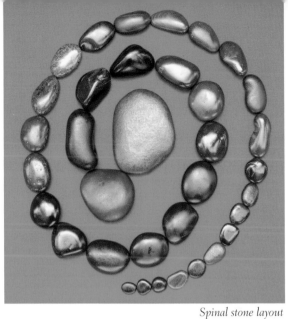

Spinal stone layout

Stone shield layout

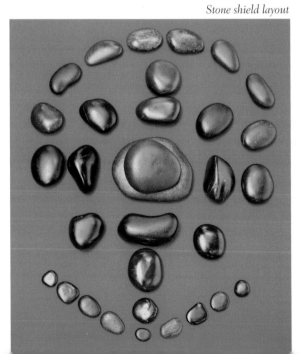

16

Basic Hot Stone Treatment

With your partner supine on a sheet-covered table.

1. To begin the treatment before the placing of any stones, start by stretching your partner. Completely stretch the legs, lower back, arms and neck. Once your partner is completely stretched and relaxed, help him or her to sit up on the table.

2. Remove the stones from the roaster. Consult the diagrams for stone placement for the back (page 55, top). Then place the stones on the table and create the spinal layout. Maker certain that the stones are on either side of the spine and are not hitting the vertebra.

   Cover the stones with two pillowcases, and gently help your partner lie down on the stones. If your partner feels any discomfort, adjust the stones.

3. Add a bolster or rolled up towel under the knees.

4. Remove the cervical stone from the roaster or ice chest and place under your partner's neck.

5. Remove two hand stones from the roaster. Fold the sheet over your partner's hands and place the stones on top of the sheet. If the stones are too hot, fold the sheet twice.

At this point, ask your partner if they are comfortable with the temperature of the stones he or she is lying on. If the stones are too hot, add another pillowcase layer.

6. Remove the sacral stone from the roaster. The sacral stone is a larger stone that has been placed in the center of the roaster. Place this stone on the table, either on the side or between your partner's legs below the knee.

7. Remove the four large effleurage stones, the third eye and throat chakra stone from the roaster. Place these next to the belly stone on the table. At this point you can add a dab of your favorite essential oil to the stones.

8. This would be a good place to present an induction (verbal visualization) for your partner. It can be something like this:

"(Name of partner), take a deep breath. Now, take a second breath and allow your body to gently sink into the stones. As you continue to breath, deeply relax. Make a connection to the stones. Allow the heat of the stones to gently penetrate your body.

Now, bring your attention back into this moment, into your body, and ask yourself, 'What do I want out of this session?' Make a mental note of it. Take another deep breath and acknowledge the elements of fire, water, air and earth. These elements have been used in preparation of this session, and they overlap with the mental, emotional, physical and spiritual bodies. Take a moment to honor yourself, and give yourself permission to fully experience this session and extract from it everything you need. Breathe deeply as you acknowledge your feelings and emotions. Ask your angels and guides to guide you during this session."

This is one example of the many ways you can do a guided visualization with your partner. Be creative, practice, and have fun.

9. To bring and maintain balance to the energy flow in the body, we must maintain the polarities that are dominant in the body. These polarities follow imaginary lines of energy from the head to the feet. These are positive and negative energies similar to a battery and, like a battery, a charge is created when connected to an outside source. To create this charge in stone massage therapy we use a technique

called Energy Connection (see diagrams on page 50).

The numbers correspond to the numbers on the diagram on page 50

❖ Hold both ankles **1** and take a deep breath and concentrate on feeling the wave of balancing energy that you can send from your hands to your partner.

❖ Slowly move your hands from the ankles to the knees. **2** Again, take a deep breath and concentrate on feeling the wave of balancing energy that you can send from your hands to your partner.

❖ Slowly move your hands from the knees to the hips. **3** Take and hold a deep breath, this time concentrating on the wave of calming and balancing energy moving from your heart and hands to your partner's body.

❖ Slowly move your hands from the hips to the shoulders. **4** Take a deep breath and allow a wave of energy to go into your partner's body.

❖ Gently move both of your hands to cradle your partner's head. **6** Take a deep breath and feel the wave of balancing energy you are sending all the way down your partner's body from the head to the feet.

Remember, when you do the energy connection in front of the body, you must do it on the back as well.

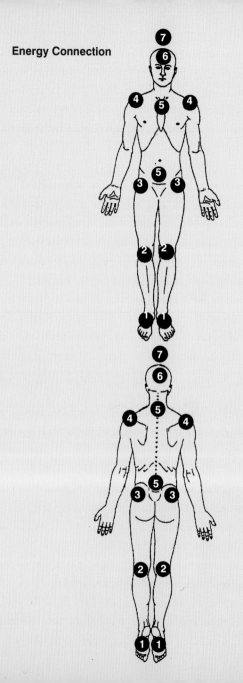

Energy Connection

10. Now you can start placing the front chakra layout stones (diagram page 50). Begin with the large stone (sacral stone). Place right above the pubic bone followed by the other four stones. Gently touch your partner's throat and third eye before placing the stones (make sure that these stones are warm, not hot).

11. Oil feet and legs. Remove the toe stones from the roaster. Place them between the feet and massage the feet with them as you place them between the toes.

12. Remove the two medium effleurage stones from the roaster and start working the right leg.

    Remember, always touch the body with the back of your hand first. The first touch should never be a hot stone. If the stones are too hot, let them cool off a minute or two before applying to the body.

    When you are finished with the leg and the stones are cool, return the stones to the roaster to reheat.

13. Remove two medium effleurage stones from the roaster and work the left leg. Then, return the stones to the roaster to reheat.

14. Remove two medium effleurage stones from the roaster and work both the right and left leg.

15. Oil the right arm. Use the hand stone your partner has been holding to work the right hand and arm.

When finished, leave that stone for your partner to hold.

16. Oil the left arm. Use the hand stone your partner has been holding to work the left hand and arm. When finished, leave that stone for your partner to hold.

17. Remove two medium effleurage stones from the roaster and work the right arm.

18. Remove two medium effleurage stones from the roaster and work the left arm.

19. Remove two medium effleurage stones from the roaster and work the right and left arms.

20. Remove the cervical, throat and third eye stones.

21. Oil the neck and shoulders.

22. Remove all neck stones from the roaster. Wrap them in a towel and use them to work the neck, upper shoulders and upper chest.

23. At this point, you can use the cold stones to work the neck and upper shoulders. You can also use the small face stones.

Remember, always let your partner know you are changing to cold stones. I usually ask my partner to take a deep breath and say, "This is going to be cool."

24. After you finish with the cold stones, you can remove the toe stones. Remove the front chakra layout stones and hand stones and return them to the roaster to reheat.

25. Help your partner to sit up, and cover his or her back with a towel. Offer your partner some water and some serenity as you silently remove the stones from the table. Don't return the spinal stones to the roaster.

With your partner prone.

26. Remove the large belly stone from the roaster. Wrap it in a pillowcase and place it on the table (illustration page 54, bottom). Ask your partner to turn over and place the belly stone anywhere there is no bone (placing the belly stone on bone such as the pubic bone, iliac crest or lower ribs will be uncomfortable).

27. I usually apply some lavender essential oil to the back. Then I do some stretching and rocking while the stones in the roaster get hot again. Generally it takes four to five minutes for the stones to reheat.

28. If you did the energy connection to the front of the body, you have to do it to the back.

29. Remove the five back chakra layout stones from the roaster (see the illustration on page 62, top). Start the layout with the large sacral stone and then the four other stones.

Stone layout for prone position

Client is draped with towel

Hot stones for front layout on top of towel, not on bare skin

Hand stones over folded sheet not on bare skin

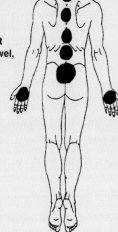

Belly stone wrapped with pillow case

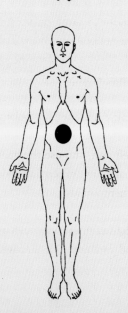

30. Bring the two hand stones out of the roaster. Fold the sheet over your partner's hands and place the stones on top of the sheet.

31. Oil the legs and buttocks.

32. Remove two medium effleurage stones from the roaster and start working the left leg. When the stones lose their heat, return them to the roaster.

33. Remove two medium effleurage stones from the roaster and start working the right leg. When the stones lose their heat, return them to the roaster.

34. Remove two medium effleurage stones from the roaster and work the left and right legs.

35. Now, remove the four upper stones from the back chakra layout and return them to the roaster to reheat. Bring the towel down, place the sacral stone back and fold the towel to expose the buttocks and back.

36. Oil the entire back and buttocks again, if necessary.

37. Oil the left arm, and use the hand stone to work the left hand and arm. When finished, leave that stone for your partner to hold.

38. Oil the right arm, and use the hand stone to work the right hand and arm. When finished, leave that stone for your partner to hold.

39. Remove two medium effleurage stones from the roaster and start working the left leg. This time you can continue to the left buttock with long effleurage strokes. Go up the shoulders and work the back.

Remember, when you are ready to replace stones, go down the arms and replace the hand stones with the two stones you have been working.

40. Remove two medium effleurage stones from the roaster and start working the right leg. Continue to the right buttock with long effleurage strokes. Go up the shoulders and work the back.

41. Remove two large effleurage stones from the roaster. Go to the left leg. Go up the body and start working the buttocks and back.

Remember, be creative and take your time. Using the stones, glide slowly with firm pressure.

42. Repeat steps 32 to 41 two to three times. Remember to replace the hand stones your partner is holding with warm stones as you finish using them.

43. Now, bring some cold stones from the ice chest and work the upper body and neck. Before applying the cold stones, ask your partner to breathe and tell him or her that "this is going to be cool."

Remember, always start the cold stones in the upper body and work down. Never hold cold stones over the kidneys for any length of time.

44. At this point you can remove the hand stones and the sacral stone. Cover your partner with a towel.

The treatment is nearly finished. You will want to provide further balance and to close the back chakra layout so that your partner is not left wide open. For this I use the Hopi Technique. This technique is based on the healing method called Healing Touch developed by Dr. Barbara Brennan. Healing Touch has been adapted from ancient healing-by-touch techniques including those by Australian Aborigines and the North American Hopi Indians. It incorporates the East Indian Chakra System as well as some ancient Chinese techniques.

45. Hopi Technique

This is done with a room temperature stone. You may use a Chinese fluorite, a quartz crystal or any other stone with a rounded or semi-pointed end.

❖ Position yourself on your partner's left side.

❖ Place your thumb and index finger on either side of your partner's spine below the neck.

❖ Hold a small stone in your right hand and begin to make nine clockwise circles in the direction of the right shoulder just underneath

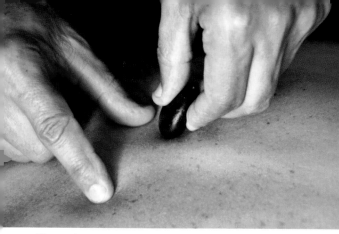

Hopi technique

your index finger. Then make nine counter-clockwise circles in the direction of the left shoulder just under your thumb.

❖ After completing each of the nine circles glide the stone down the side of the body as far as you can go.

❖ When this step is completed move your fingers down approximately 2" (5cm) and repeat the sequence again.

❖ Continue like this until you get all the way down to the sacrum (the large bone at the end of the spine at the bottom of the lower back).

The nine clockwise circles represent spirit, and the nine counterclockwise circles represent rebirth. This brings a wonderful awareness and balance to the close of the session.

46. If you own a Tibetan singing bowl, this is the time to use it. Place the bowl between your partner's shoulder blades and gently hit the bowl four times.

Tibetan singing bowls have been made for more than 2,500 years. They can be referred to as standing bells since they are meant to be struck while sitting on a surface rather than hung like a standard bell. Their sound promotes a deep sense of relaxation, and singing bowls are useful in meditation. Contemporary versions are available through many internet sources.

47. Wash your partner's feet and hands with something cool and refreshing such as witch hazel, which I prefer, or alcohol. For an extra touch, add a few drops of peppermint oil.

48. Walk to the top of the table, put your hand on your partner's upper back and say something like, "The session has come to an end. Very gently bring your awareness back to the room."

49. Don't forget to say, "Thank you."   *Tibetan singing bowl*

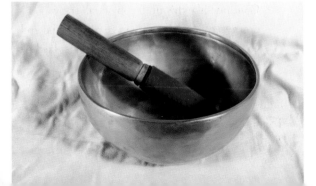

17

Additional Stone Layouts

❖ Front Chakra Layout (see opposite)

❖ Spinal Layout (page 20)

❖ Back Chakra Layout (page 62)

Stone layout for supine position

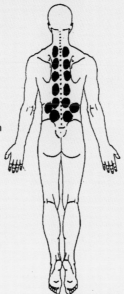

Hot stones for back layout are covered with two pillowcases before the client lies down on them

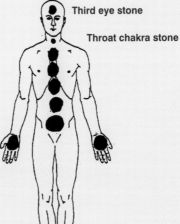

Third eye stone

Five chakra stones on top of towel, not on bare skin

Throat chakra stone

Hand stones over folded sheet not on bare skin

Client is draped with towel

Warm toe stones

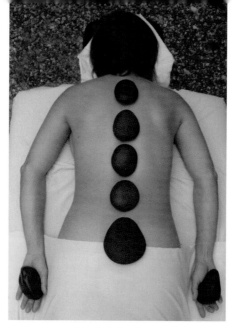

Back chakra layout

Energy circle for lower mid back, stomach, and solar plexus

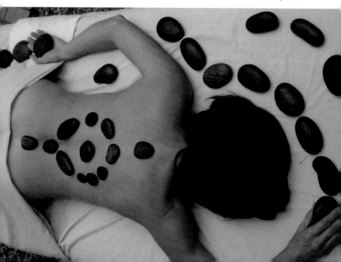

18

House Calls

WHILE IT MAY BE DIFFICULT TO DO FULL BODY treatments on a house call, partial treatments are possible. You'll want a smaller, more portable 9 to 10 quart (8.5L to 9.5L) roaster and a smaller set of stones (preferably 10 in number) in addition to your folding massage table.

Everything (except the massage table) should fit into a gym bag. Include an extension cord, wooden spoon, thermometer and two hand towels. Your partner should provide a large towel to place under the roaster, and a solid surface on which to place the roaster.

Begin your setup with the roaster so that the stones can be heating up while you arrange everything else. By the time your partner gets to the table, the stones should be at the right temperature (130°F to 140°F/55°C to 60°C).

If you start with cold water, keep in mind that it will take approximately 20 minutes for the water to reach 135°F (57°C). If you start with hot water from the tap, it will take approximately 10 minutes for the water to reach that temperature.

Once the stones are ready, you're ready to go!

About the Author

Ernesto Ortiz, LMT, CST, KRM, is the founder and director of *Journey to the Heart*, a company dedicated to the raising of consciousness and the well-being of people. He is a noted artist and author; a renowned and inspiring facilitator, teacher and therapist; and is recognized for his innovative, explorative, and multi-dimensional training in massage therapy, CranioSacral therapy, Karmapa Reiki, Integrative/Shamanic techniques, Breathwork, Akashic Records, music therapy, and Trance Dance. His training started at an early age with Shamans and Curanderos in Mexico and South America and has continued with teachers from all over the world.

Ernesto has devoted his life to exploring and communicating the language of the heart, primal movement and deep inner spaces. Over the past 25 years, he has taken thousands of people on a journey from physical and emotional inertia to the freedom of ecstasy, from the chaos of the chattering ego-mind to the blessed emptiness of stillness and inner silence.

His Workshops and Retreats have an electric intensity that unifies the spiritual with the mundane, from the poetic discovery of the soul to the modern approach of ancient shamanic practices. He has facilitated numerous workshops and seminars in the US, Canada, Australia, the Caribbean, Indonesia, Egypt, the UK and South America.

Ernesto is the author of *In the Presence of Love* and *Mastering the Art of Relationships*, among others. His Akashic Records and Tian Di Bamboo workshop are also available on DVD. For more information visit www.journey2theheart.com.